HOW TO BLITZ NITS
(AND OTHER NASTIES)

HOW TO BLITZ NITS
(AND OTHER NASTIES)

Written By
IONA BOWER

Edited by
JUSTINE ROBERTS

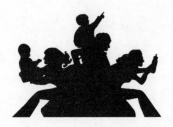

BLOOMSBURY
LONDON · OXFORD · NEW YORK · NEW DELHI · SYDNEY

Bloomsbury Publishing
An imprint of Bloomsbury Publishing Plc

50 Bedford Square   1385 Broadway
London   New York
WC1B 3DP   NY 10018
UK   USA

www.bloomsbury.com

BLOOMSBURY and the Diana logo are trademarks of Bloomsbury Publishing Plc

First published in Great Britain 2017

© Mumsnet Limited, 2017
Illustrations by Paul Boston

Mumsnet Limited has asserted its right under the Copyright, Designs and Patents
Act, 1988, to be identified as Author of this work.

British Library Cataloguing-in-Publication Data
A catalogue record for this book is available from the British Library.

Library of Congress Cataloguing-in-Publication data has been applied for.

ISBN: HB: 978-1-4088-6215-5
ePub: 978-1-4088-6216-2

2 4 6 8 10 9 7 5 3 1

Typeset by Newgen Knowledge Works Pvt Ltd., Chennai, India
Printed and bound in Great Britain by CPI Group (UK) Ltd, Croydon CR0 4YY

For every Mumsnetter who has valiantly entered into battle with nits (and other nasties) and lived to tell the tale.

Contents

Introduction   1
Nits   9
Threadworms   21
Ringworm   35
Warts and Verrucas   47
Molluscum   59
Conjunctivitis   71
Foreign Objects   83
Vomit   95
Poo   109
Dragons under the Bed   121
Postscript   135

Introduction

(Please leave your decorousness at the door)

Raising children, it turns out, is basically an extreme form of pest control. Pre-children, you probably imagined that a goodly portion of parenthood would involve teaching them to listen to the sea in a shell, sewing tiny ladybird buttons onto pinafore dresses and stroking warm little backs bundled up in sleeping bags in the semi-dark. How wrong we all were.

Seeing your offspring safely through from birth to 'Isn't it time you got your own place now, sweetheart?' can, in practice, take on the character of a dogged slog through one horror after another, from fungus to phobia, parasite to plague, excretion to emesis. In any given week, if they haven't succumbed to a vomiting bug, the chances are they'll have picked up nits or threadworms. When you finally manage to see off the wart that's been squatting on their hand for a year, you'll notice a lovely patch of ringworm blooming on the other arm. And that's before you take into account the beasties your child will invite in all of their own accord, from dragons under the bed invading their mind and your sleep to Lego lightsabers inserted deftly up the nostril.

In short, your child's body can feel like a battle-ground of nasty little pests, particularly during the nursery and school years, when regiments of lice, threadworms, common colds and tummy bugs keep up a constant vigil, seeking out the small, the weak, the long of hair and the sucky of thumb to make good their entrance. Welcome to the jungle.

Face down your foe

Every parent will of course have their own particular nemesis – the childhood nasty they dread above all others. There are those who take a sanguine approach to parasites such as head lice and threadworms, while others, when faced with the same, seriously consider moving their child into the shed and leaving them provisions in a vinegar stone, plague-village-style. As one Mumsnetter told her talk board comrades:

'I DETEST parasites of any sort. Apparently more than 70% of living things on the earth are actually parasites. Nice huh?'

SamuelWestsMistress

Some of us, meanwhile, feel light-headed at the thought of having to retrieve a snot-covered mouldy pea from inside a nostril, while others take it in their stride, as this traumatised soul testified:

'One of the most disgusting things I have ever seen was a toddler in a pram at the traffic lights who did a massive "snot sneeze". His mum just leaned forward and slurped all the snot up; she didn't even spit it out. My mum and I just stood there open-mouthed. We missed the green man and everything. My mum called weakly after her, "I had a tissue."'

Notso

Considering carefully which particular horror you dread most, however, will get us nowhere. When all's said and done, it's about context:

'Which is worse, nits or threadworms? Answer: whichever one is in YOUR house RIGHT NOW.'

Bogeyface

Wise words indeed. It's time to buckle up, knuckle down, and get your hands dirty.

Bring out the big guns (or large gins)
Of course, some fights are harder-won than others. Should you be exceedingly unlucky, you may find yourself battling a war on two fronts, in which more than one 'nasty' needs nixing at once:

> 'It was when we all had threadworms and nits at the same time that I knew I had truly arrived as a parent.'
>
> *Foxinsocks*

Solutions there may be to all manner of pest and plague, but there's a time and a place, too, for drowning your sorrows in a large drink, or six cubic feet of chocolate. If you've given everything a go and your child and home are still infested with whichever nightmare being you were seeking to evict, well, there's succour to be found in drowning your sorrows, and comfort to be taken from the knowledge that someone, somewhere, has had it worse than you and lived to tell the tale. A moment of respectful silence, please, for this poor Mumsnetter and her dramatic brush with bodily fluids.

'I turn off the tap to the bath that I am filling for us to share. THUD. A turd the size of a corn on the cob drops from his tiny peach of a bum onto my landing carpet... I wrestle the monster into the toilet and clean my son up.

Son: "I've done another poo in my bedroom." There is diarrhoea smeared all over his bedroom carpet. I clean it up, pop him in the bath, and get in myself. Have just wet my hair with a cup when my son smiles and announces he has done a big wee in the bath and then... vomits on me. TWICE.

So I'm sitting with piss dripping from my hair, raisins stuck to my tits and yoghurt floating around me. I wearily get up, put on the shower and pull out the plug. I'm shoving bits of food down the plug hole with my big toe while cleaning us both off...

Next day, I found a five pound note on the ground. Normally I'd ask around in case anyone had dropped it but I shoved it into my pocket in the firm belief that it had been sent down from God himself as if to say, "Go on girl, treat yourself. I sent you all kinds of crap yesterday, get yourself something nice."'

Donbean

It's true that you have to take your breaks where you can find them as a parent. But while succour and support have their place, what moments like these call for are the quick wits and clear thinking of those who have been there before.

Call in the cavalry
Unfortunately, no one's going to bail you out of any of these battles. You were press-ganged unknowingly the day that thin blue line appeared, and now you're foot soldier, firefighter and Chief of Defence Staff rolled into one.

That's the bad news. The good news is that there's help and advice at hand from an army of individuals who've been in the same boat. Since the dawn of time, parents have been disinfecting riddled hair, scraping bodily fluids off clothes and turfing out monsters, both real and imaginary, from their homes. And in more modern times, they've very kindly shared their solutions on Mumsnet.

In this book, we've addressed ten of the most common childhood nasties and scoured the Mumsnet talk boards (a.k.a. the coalface) for the simplest, most ingenious and amusing cures. Some come with an NHS seal of approval, others are very definitely from the 'old wives' school of medicine (in fact, many are entirely without medical or scientific recommendation, so we do advise you to approach them with caution and entirely at your own risk) – but crucially, all of them have worked for *someone* out there.

Grit your teeth, gird your loins and get the freezer jacket on the wine bottle. This is not the end. It is not even the beginning of the end. But it might just be the end of the beginning. . . Until the next attack.

Nits

(How to keep your head when all
around you are scratching theirs. . .)

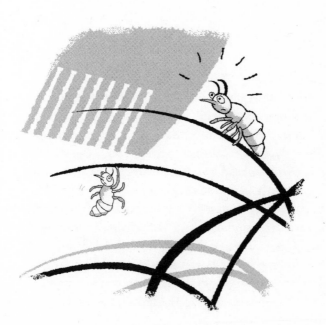

It begins with a note in your child's bag. 'We have nits in school,' it announces, breezily, as if informing you of the date of the Christmas concert. In fact, as every parent knows, the phrase is spin for 'burn your bedding, paint a plague cross on your door and prepare for the apocalypse'.

But there is hope. Keep your cool and you can win – and rebuild, once the war is over. Here's how to nix a nit without surrendering your sanity.

KNOW YOUR ENEMY

HEAD LOUSE (*pediculis humanus capitis*)
Thought to have originated in North America – though nit shells have been found on mummies. Nits are the small, white eggs, lice the fully-grown adults: greyish, about the size of a sesame seed, with six clawed legs and sharp mouth-parts for sucking blood (yours). The adults lay their eggs on the hair shaft in warm spots (behind ears and at the nape of the neck). Once hatched, the lice are capable of reproducing in six to ten days. The females lay on average five eggs a day, so the little buggers multiply at an alarming rate.

STRENGTH: 4

Their strength is in numbers. Harmless, but *extremely* annoying.

AGILITY: 1

Head lice don't have wings and can't jump, so are reduced to crawling from head to head. On paper, that sounds tricky, but like all creatures that exist under the law of sod, they manage it. On the plus side, there's no chance of them leaping at you, face-hugger style.

SKILLS: 4

Blood-sucking, speed-mating, interbreeding. Like a bad boyfriend, basically.

SPEED: 1

A head louse can travel approximately 23cm a minute. Easily outpaced.

INTELLIGENCE: 2

Not going to impress on *University Challenge*, but fast becoming immune to many nit treatments.

ACHILLES HEEL

Fine-toothed combs.

Assemble your arsenal

Preparation is all. Don't wait for the note; accept the fact that, at some point during their educational career your children will be infested, and hit your nearest chemist to stock up. If you've got the basics (a nit comb – the queen of which is the Nitty Gritty – and a bottle of conditioner), you'll be able to swing into action as soon as the enemy makes landfall.

Begin manoeuvres

When you receive the dreaded letter – or if you spot your child scratching – act fast. Wash their hair, rinse, apply lots of conditioner and leave on. Use a wide-toothed comb to detangle, then get to work with your Nitty Gritty. Separate the hair into sections and work through individually, comb-ing carefully from roots to tips and inspecting the comb for squatters each time. Wipe the comb on a tissue or rinse in a bowl of water with each sweep, so you can see what you've netted.

> 'Don't waste your money on lice shampoos. The only way to get rid of lice is to comb and comb and comb.'
>
> Sofia Ames

It can take hours (that feel like weeks) to comb through your child's hair, especially if it's long – but

it is, on the plus side, a job with high satisfaction
levels:

> 'One day I got almost 100 eggs out of my
> daughter's hair. I had a pot of hot water that
> I dipped the comb in after each pass, and it
> looked like Wembley Stadium by the time I was
> done! I really enjoy sending them to their scald-
> ing death.'
>
>   Minimou

Roll out the big guns

If you find live lice, rather than just nits, use a head
lice treatment. These fall into two camps: Poison-
Them-and-Suffocate-Them-and-Slide-Them-Off.

You'll probably remember the nit treatments of
your youth. They were basically DDT: a heavy-duty
insecticide which did the job but didn't make for a
pleasant experience. You can still buy the stuff, but the
problem (beyond your child's streaming eyes) is that
the lice have developed immunity to it (a US study
found that lice in 25 of 30 states studied were invul-
nerable). The alternatives, more popular these days,
are silicone- or oil-based, and work by either dehy-
drating the lice or smothering them in goo (which,
conveniently, makes them easier to remove).

Whichever method you choose, you'll still need
to comb afterwards. Some treatments claim only

to need one application, after which lice and eggs can be brushed out – but the combing method, though painstaking, is the only way to know for certain you've got them all. And remember, it's not enough to get rid of the lice; the eggs must go, too, or you'll be back to square one within a week. Thoroughness is key.

Alternative options

If you don't fancy the over-the-counter treatments (or, indeed, if you've been through the whole shelf and STILL haven't emerged victorious), there are other options.

The only natural repellent proven to have an effect is tea tree, but there's plenty of anecdotal evidence for other solutions, from gently discouraging with lavender oil to zapping with electric nit combs. Thrill-seekers may be attracted by the various frying methods. . .

'After treatment and combing, and once hair is dry, use a hair straightener to completely cook them. Worked really well on my daughter!'

Sev

'A vote for the electronic comb: very effective, and it was satisfying knowing that every time the buzz changed you'd zapped one of the buggers.'

Nennypops

. . . while those of a milder bent might prefer aromatherapy.

'Neem oil: it's foul-smelling and nits HATE it. I can guarantee it will work.'

AlwaysCheerful

'I make my own mix: base oil with drops of tea tree, eucalyptus and geranium. No nit has been known to survive.'

QuintessentialShadows

Still others turn to the kitchen cupboard:

'My mum swore by neat malt vinegar. She'd tip a massive bottle in the sink and dunk our heads. Christ, it stung if you got it in your eye, but all the lice just jumped off! Next day she did the same and that was it. All dead.'

SparkleToffee

'Wine or cider vinegar as a final rinse, left on the hair and then blow-dried. Do it on a Friday, though, as your child will smell like a chip shop.

> Apparently, a comb-through with strong alcohol
> (e.g. vodka) works, too.'
>
> BurberryQ

(To clarify: that's vodka for combing through the hair, rather than for drinking while you're combing. But whatever works, obviously.)

The other key method involves depriving the blighters of oxygen. Veterans will regale you with tales of killing nits by covering their child's hair in mayonnaise, slapping a shower cap on, sending them to bed and washing it out in the morning. This method is precisely as foul as it sounds, but if your infestation is of long standing, it may seem a small price to pay. And if all else fails? Call the vet.

> 'A friend who's a vet uses Frontline on his children to keep away nits. Apparently it's very effective.'
>
> QuietTiger

No kidding. . .

Clearing the battlefield

Let one thing be understood: head lice are persistent. So you've made your first pass; think you can sit back and crack open the gin? Think again. Now is the time to consolidate. Once you've Nitty

Gritty-ed, you should repeat on days three, six, nine, twelve and fifteen. We recommend a child-friendly DVD box set to get you through.

Head lice can live only on humans, so pets will remain unmolested, but you DO need to check everyone else in the household for infestation. Under-tens tend to be most vulnerable, but don't for a moment assume anyone is immune.

> 'My son last got them when he was four-teen. Fourteen! I was moved to ask him what exactly he was doing that was taking him into such close contact with Heads With Nasties.'
>
> *Shodan*

Bedding, toys and clothes should be put through as hot a wash as possible; a quick spin at thirty degrees is the equivalent of a lice spa-day. Brushes, combs, bands and so forth should be soaked in boiling water. If that feels insufficient, chuck the lot away and start over. You are, after all, worth it.

Establishing defences

Congratulations: you've won the opening bat-tle. Now's the time to step back and consider the war. Firstly, reduce the risk of acquisition by tying back long hair. A nice, tight plait, secured at each end, is the Mumsnet-preferred option. You ever see Princess Elsa with nits? Nope.

There are various things you can apply to hair that are anecdotally effective. Many Mumsnetters swear by Vosene shampoo. Tea tree oil, mixed with water and spritzed, is said to be a repellent; ditto lavender oil. And apparently, hair gel makes it harder for the lice to attach their eggs – so long as you don't mind sending your boys to school looking like a Bros tribute band. If it doesn't work, it will at least keep you amused until they get fed up with it.

'My hairdresser says to use tea tree oil in shampoo to prevent head lice, and also to send them to school with a little bit of gel or spray on their hair to help prevent lice from gripping the hair.'

Gemtubbs

If you want to get out in front of the problem, pick a time each week (Sunday nights are popular, since they're awful already) and get combing. Think of it as part of your end-of-week ritual, like shoe-polishing, or *Antiques Roadshow*.

'Nit Sunday: weekly washing and conditioning and going through with a nit comb. Better than any medication. If you find any evidence then do more frequently; every day if bad for a few days, then back to once a week. Works for us.'

SparkleRainbow

Finally, there are those apocryphal parents who, in the face of infestation, shave their children's heads. This will work, as long as you can cope with the sobbing, the reactions of others, and the redundancy of your arsenal of Peppa Pig hair-bands.

Frankly, though, you can buy every preparation on the market, send your child to school in a swimming cap and make a pact with Satan, but you might well end up with nits anyway. Along with death and taxes, if you have children, head lice are one of life's certainties.

'With head lice, I went for all-out war on the little feckers. Deterrent spray. Nitty Gritty and conditioner every hair wash. Electronic zappy comb on returning home from school. And my daughter STILL caught them. After nuclear war, the only things that will survive are cockroaches and head lice.'

Droves

Keep calm and carry on combing.

AMAZING NIT FACT

A female head louse has to mate only once to pro-
duce all her eggs. After that she stores sperm in her
body, releasing it when needed, thus avoiding the
human conundrum of how to conceive number
two when you've not had more than four con-
secutive hours' sleep for years. . .

Threadworms

(Why every parent needs a headlamp in their medicine cabinet)

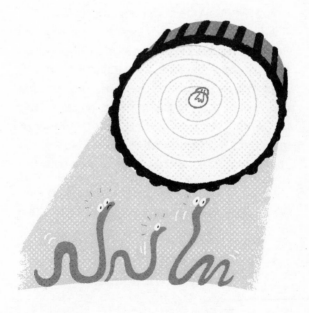

There's no prettying up a threadworm. Firstly, it's a worm. Secondly, it's made its home up your child's bottom. And finally, and most insultingly, once there, it absorbs nutrients from their body. Remember that broccoli pasta you lovingly prepared? Threadworms have had that away. Angry now? You should be. Without further ado, here's the definitive guide on how to repel the parasite that taste forgot. . .

KNOW YOUR ENEMY

THREADWORM (*enterobius vermicularis*)
Evidence of threadworms exists as far back as 7800 BC; they even get a mention by Hippocrates. Tiny parasites that live in the gut and emerge at night to lay eggs around the anus, they look like small, white threads and measure between 2mm and 13mm. They mostly affect children under ten; in fact, it's estimated that around 40% (yes!) of under-tens have threadworms at any one time.

STRENGTH: 1
The females die after laying eggs, so at least they aren't perennial.

AGILITY: 1
No legs, so fairly limited.

SKILLS: 5
Making and excreting their own glue. Useful at
any craft session.

SPEED: 0
Paula Radcliffe has nothing to fear.

INTELLIGENCE: 1
Smart enough to emerge only at night; otherwise,
little promise academically.

ACHILLES HEEL
Carrot and garlic salad.

How did they get. . . you know. . . up there?
Your child ate them. Sorry. Child A has worms, scratches bottom, collects eggs under fingernails, transfers them to Play-Doh/sandpit/book. Child B handles said object, picks up eggs on fingers, sticks fingers in mouth. Swallowed eggs travel to the intestine, hatch, and are fully grown within two weeks. Worms pop out at night to lay eggs around the anus, and the whole miraculous cycle begins again. Jolly good.

Informing the landlord

> 'They're not so bad. I used to think of them as annoying, temporary lodgers.'
>
> *Hiddenhome*

If your child is young, you may choose to avoid full disclosure. A simple 'this medicine will clear up your itchy bum' raises fewer questions than 'there are several hundred worms up your behind, scoffing your dinner and waiting until you're asleep to crawl out.' Anthropomorphise as little as possible; it won't help anyone.

On the other hand, older children, who thrive on the yuck factor, may be intrigued. A rousing chorus of 'there's a worm at the bottom of your colon, and his name is Wiggly Woo' will keep spirits up. However, avoid the 'think of it as a pet' route, or you'll have tears when a thousand wormy corpses fall into the toilet bowl. Stick to the bare facts. They're impressive enough.

'My son had worms a few weeks ago. Yesterday he saw an earthworm on the pavement and asked what it was. "A worm," I said. "I wonder whose bottom it fell out of," he replied.'

DeWe

Spotting the squatters
The key sign that you're hosting uninvited guests is itching – caused not by the worms but the 'glue' they use to stick their eggs around the anus. If you spot your child scratching (more than usual) it's worth investigating. Worms can make their way to the vagina, too, so if little girls complain of itching in that area, worms are a possibility. If you suspect worms, have a good look. Yes, up there.

'If mine say they have an itchy bottom and I can't see anything I tell them to "pretend to push a poo" – then often you'll see one just inside.'

Unlucky83

There's a rather obvious hazard with this, so do stand well back.

In borderline cases, many parents choose to err on the side of caution and worm everyone in the house, but if you need proof, there are a few more methods for diagnosis:

The Shitty Stick Test

- Apparatus: Stick, potty, strong stomach.
- Method: If your parenting experience thus far has not called for raking through poo, brace yourself. A bit of bamboo cane is ideal for the job: not so long as to be unwieldy nor so short as to risk accidentally dipping a sleeve.
- Results: Accurate – but you might wish you'd just trusted your instincts.

The Blue Peter Test

- Apparatus: Sellotape, slide from the GP, brass neck.
- Method: Apply a piece of sticky tape over the anus first thing in the morning. Peel away and stick on the slide; give the slide to your GP to send off to the lab.
- Results: The only way to get a definitive diagnosis – but you may get 'a look' if you go into your practice waving the Sellotape and demanding tests. Your GP will usually

suggest that if you suspect worms it's fine to go ahead and treat for it.

The Arthur Scargill Test

- Apparatus: Miner's helmet (or torch, if you can't lay your hands on one); cover of darkness.
- Method: Sneak into your sleeping child's bedroom. Grip the torch between your teeth, peel back pyjama bottoms and look to see if there are any worms waving back at you. Expect them to have a rabbit-in-headlights look in their eyes.
- Results: Works well, but if your child wakes, you might have to fork out for therapy later.

In summary, if you suspect worms, it's much less traumatic to treat everyone in the family than seek out a diagnosis. No method of checking is 100% foolproof and you might be wasting valuable hours of your life that could be spent – well, doing anything else, really.

The eviction process

To nail those little bastards, you need to do it properly. This involves a two-pronged attack.

Part one: Treat everyone in the house
Unless one of you is pregnant, breastfeeding, or under two, you don't need to go to your GP; you can buy worming treatments over the counter at the pharmacy. The most common are those containing mebendazole (e.g. Ovex), which works by preventing the worms from absorbing glucose, which eventually starves them.

If you were dosed with Pripsen and are concerned that your child, too, will never again look a raspberry milkshake in the eye, fear not: modern treatments don't taste nearly as bad as those you remember.

> 'It's a family legend that we children were moaning about the taste of Pripsen, and my dad said something no-nonsense like "oh it can't be that bad, just get on with it", then took his, went purple, gagged, swore, and announced he'd never tasted anything as vile in all his born days, and we must all have chocolate immediately.'
>
> **Puddock**

Happily, Ovex is available in an orange-flavoured chewy tablet or a banana-flavoured suspension fluid. It's not going to make it onto *The Great British*

Menu, but it's far less likely to induce nausea than the treatments of days gone by.

Part two: Launch a hygiene offensive
The treatment kills only the worms, not the eggs, so you need to wash them away. Approach this with a forensic level of care. You're gonna wash those parasites right outta your house. Here's how:

DAY ONE: DEEP CLEAN

1. Wash all bedding, towels and cuddly toys on a hot wash. There may be tears but unless you want your child inhaling worm eggs off Mr Rabbit, you're going to have to tough this one out.
2. Vacuum thoroughly, especially in bedrooms and anywhere people remove clothes. Change the Hoover bag afterwards, outside and with care.
3. Dust, using a damp cloth so that the eggs stick to the cloth and you aren't simply moving them around, especially in the bathroom and kitchen. Plunge the cloths you use into hot water regularly while cleaning and bin them all after use. Replace toothbrushes and keep them in a closed cupboard.

FOR TWO WEEKS AFTER TAKING THE MEDICATION AND THE DEEP CLEAN

1. Everyone should wear close-fitting underwear in bed. Help little ones take pants off carefully so any eggs don't get shaken onto the floor and put straight in the washing machine. If possible, get your children to wear cotton gloves in bed, so if they scratch, they don't get eggs stuck under their fingernails. Give it the old Princess Elsa spiel ('Conceal, don't feel') if they're not keen.
2. Change nightwear daily.
3. Each morning, stand them in the bath and wash away any eggs that have been laid overnight.

'Make sure the family takes off underwear and places it gently and immediately in a laundry basket. (No flinging, no waving around, no wearing on the head.) Keep the laundry basket in the bathroom and make everyone undress there. The bathroom floor should be hosed down daily.'

Mathanxiety

If worms are still in evidence, you can do another dose after two weeks to hoover up hangers-on. It's perfectly reasonable at this point to scream: 'Die, bastards, die!' as you administer the medication.

'Outside the box' methods of eviction
Many swear by comestible warfare, though we would caution against some of the methods that seem to have been used by Mumsnetters' own mothers.

> 'I'm an eighties child of a hippy mother. I remember her shoving a clove of garlic up mine and my sisters' bums like a suppository. Oh, how we screamed. No idea if it worked or not.'
>
> *Bellaoftheballs*

> 'My parents' 1980s cure for worms was to soak raisins in brandy then make us swallow them whole! Dunno if it worked, but I don't seem to have worms now.'
>
> *Suedeeffectpochete*

On a less dramatic note, threadworms allegedly hate raw carrot: try grating some up and giving it to your child first thing each morning. And it seems the garlic thing works if you eat it, too: grate garlic into oil then drizzle onto salad and pasta, or mix it with natural yoghurt and grated cucumber. Give them carrot sticks to dip and you'll have a doubly anti-wormy meal. Apparently coconut and pineapple are anathema too (presumably why you never see a worm with a pina colada).

Some parents eliminate sugar from their child's diet during an invasion, on the basis that worms need to absorb sugar to survive. There's limited evidence to support this but it won't do any harm.

Herbal remedies, such as grapefruit seed extract (Citricidal), are popular, too, though whether it's genuinely kryptonite or just so hideous it forces them out is debatable:

> 'Medicines which sneakily try to jolly them-
> selves up by feebly attempting to disguise their
> ghastliness by tasting of raspberry or whatever
> are annoying. It NEVER works. At least you
> know where you are with Citricidal. It's nasty
> and proud of it.'
>
> Clownsleftjokersright

Preventative measures
Since prevention is better than cure (and doesn't involve going on poo patrol or deep-cleaning your house), here are a few ways to help your kids dodge threadworms.

1. Keep nails short so they can't so easily get eggs stuck under them.

'If you get your kids to scrub under their nails when they come home from school, you should reduce the likelihood of them picking them up.'

Miaou

2. Try to stop them putting fingers in their noses and mouths. Nose-pickers and thumb-suckers are at particular risk.

'My son is a nose-picker. And, I hate to say, an eater. No wonder he keeps bloody getting them. . . I need a bulldog clip for his nose, bitter varnish to stop the nail biting and a cork up his bum. Hooray!!'

MrsMerton

AMAZING THREADWORM FACT
A female can lay up to 15,000 eggs, after which she dies. Understandable after all that effort.

Ringworm

(When is a worm not a worm?)

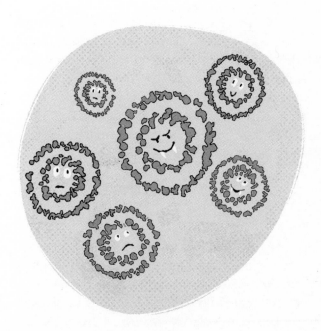

The first and most important thing you need to know about ringworm is that it's not actually a worm – it's a fungus. Obviously, as good news goes, that's a bit like hearing 'Don't worry, your house *has* burned down but we managed to save your husband's entire collection of Northern Soul on vinyl.' Still, if you'd been imagining a circular worm living under your child's skin (or, worse, a group of worms in a circle formation, synchronised swimmer-style) this will hopefully come as a relief.

In fact, ringworm is the playground bully of childhood nasties. There's one in nearly every school, it feeds on humiliation, it's not as fearsome as it sounds, and (we didn't say this) one firm punch in the kisser often sees it off for good. Here's what you need to know about The Worm That Turned (out to be nothing much to worry about in the end).

KNOW YOUR ENEMY

RINGWORM (*tinea corporis*)
Taking the 'fun' out of 'fungi' for several centuries, this fungal infection was at its height in the 1880s, particularly among the poorer classes. Nowadays it's less discriminating: any warm, damp crevice in a storm, basically. It

manifests as small patches of red on the skin. The edge of the circle is redder than the centre and sometimes more inflamed. Some people just have a single patch, others several. It tends to spring up on arms, legs and the trunk and spread from there.

STRENGTH: 3

With the correct weaponry, you'll defeat this one in two to four weeks. That said, ringworm is no weed. In fact, it regularly affects wrestlers, due to their sweaty nature. Hulk Hogan himself quakes before this fungus.

AGILITY: 3

Moves freely around the body and transfers from human to human in a single bound (or on damp towels). It's spread by touching the infected skin or other infected objects.

SKILLS: 4

Cross-breed travel. Like all playground thugs, ringworm can be found loitering around the changing rooms among the used towels. Unlike playground thugs, it also hangs out on hamsters. Yes: ringworm can actually be caught from pets – cats, dogs and guinea pigs are all prime suspects.

SPEED: 2

Though it is, in a literal sense, static, ringworm
is stealthy. Having spread its spores to another
host, it lies dormant for a few days before making
itself known.

INTELLIGENCE: 0

It's a mushroom. Need we say more?

ACHILLES HEEL

Good hygiene.

Ringworm 'on location'

For the most part, ringworm affects the trunk and face. However, it's a sneaky little fungus, and occasionally arrives elsewhere – most commonly on your feet, in which case it goes by the name athlete's foot. The 'athlete' part is a bit of a misnomer – it's called that as it tends to thrive somewhere sweaty (i.e. on feet inside trainers, post-run), but even the most sofa-bound of children can pick it up. It's common in soap-dodging, anti-sock-washing teens but is easily picked up anywhere where children go barefoot. Keep feet clean and dry and make sure socks remain on to avoid spreading it. Treat with a topical cream from the pharmacist. You shouldn't have to visit the GP unless it's persistent or spreads.

Now: if you thought fungal feet were bad, wait till you have to deal with a fungal groin. Ringworm here is fondly known as 'Jock Itch', which makes it sound like the anti-hero of a teen novel. Usually, it develops as a result of warm, moist conditions (shudder) rather than being 'caught' (phew). It appears around the genitals or inner thighs, and tends to crop up more in summer. It's worth having a brief word with the afflicted child about how to wash carefully (i.e. 'more than a quick flick with the flannel, please') and make sure they know to dry the area thoroughly. Any antifungal treatment (cream, powder or spray) from the chemist's should speed it on its way out the door.

> 'Someone I know had a fungal bottom – ugh – fixed by suppositories. Ringworm sounds like Dickensian squalor, but it is alive and well on the best of us.'
>
> Stleger

The one to really watch out for, though, is ringworm of the scalp. If it migrates up here it's harder to shift as it gets inside the hair follicles and can lead to patches of hair loss. It mostly affects children pre-puberty as the oils on the hair that arrive with teenage hormones seem to ward it off. If you suspect your child has it, you need to see your GP: it requires oral medication to shift it as well as a treatment shampoo. Chuck out their hairbrushes and accessories, and ensure they don't share towels.

Going into battle

For a generic case of ringworm, your pharmacist should be able to sort you out. Some parents prefer the certainty of a GP diagnosis, but it's always worth trying the pharmacist in the first instance in case it saves you a trip. They'll usually give you a topical ointment such as Clotrimazole, which you apply two or three times a day and then for at least two weeks after the ringworm seems to have cleared up. In particularly virulent cases, a cream that contains steroids might be prescribed by your GP.

'My son caught ringworm (from my husband, no less, who had persistent athlete's foot that he'd tried, unsuccessfully, to treat with a variety of bonkers home remedies). I popped to the GP to check it was ringworm, and she prescribed an antifungal with steroids. I wasn't keen on using a steroid cream on a young child (and the pharmacist agreed), so I bought a version of the cream but without the steroid. We applied it religiously morning and night for two weeks, and continued for another ten days after the ringworm had disappeared (this is the important bit), and it's stayed gone. As did my husband's "incurable" athlete's foot, once he'd treated it properly.'

Middlechicken

Many people find that one particular cream works for their child where others don't, so if it's not clearing up, do go back and ask for something else/stronger/more destructive.

'Lamisil AT 1% gel specifically for ringworm was prescribed by a doctor and cleared up what the Canesten didn't shift.'

Seona 1973

Arm your child for the fight

There's no doubt the best cure is a decent antifungal, but there's nothing wrong with throwing your entire arsenal at it. Keeping your child's immune system in tip-top condition will help them fight the fungus off – immune-boosting foods such as onions and garlic help ward off infections and orange veg such as squash, which tend to contain lots of vitamin A, improve skin cell renewal. Keep zinc levels high, too, with zinc-rich foods such as red meat, poultry, shellfish, wholegrains and cereals.

Unconventional weapons

If you prefer to give something milder a go before the antifungals, there are a few natural remedies you can try before trudging to the GP for a hardcore cream (or a blunderbuss). Note that these are only for use on the body or feet, not the scalp or groin.

Tea tree oil

Good old tea tree oil. It seems to cure everything from nits to a tantrum, doesn't it? Try a couple of drops in a teaspoon of carrier oil, dabbed on with a cotton bud three times a day.

Apple cider vinegar

Unproven, but your nan swears by it. Vinegar is a mild disinfectant, so this is a good solution if you have a baby with ringworm and want to try a more gentle approach. Soak a piece of folded kitchen towel in it and hold to the affected area for 15 minutes twice a day, or as often as you can.

Garlic

The tea tree oil of the food world. Crush and mix with a little olive oil, apply to the skin, put a plaster over the top and leave it for an hour or so. A word of caution: garlic can irritate, so perhaps best avoided with small children or those with sensitive skin. Don't leave it on too long either, or the skin will start to feel 'burned' (and your child will smell like Pizza Express).

Salt and vinegar

Not just an excellent pairing on chips, salt and vinegar can help see off ringworm, too. Mix one part salt to two parts apple cider vinegar and stir until it forms a paste. Apply to the skin, covering the ringworm patch, leave for five minutes, then wash off. Repeat every day for a week.

And finally...

If your kids are going to pick up only one nasty during childhood, ringworm is the one you want: not too painful; easy to treat; doesn't require you to keep them off school and meticulously clean every area of your home. The main downside is the reaction of other (dafter) parents, who may squeal and recoil in horror.

> 'I felt totally embarrassed and dirty about it. Especially after I took my son to a coffee morning. I was there five minutes and left after a chorus of "it's highly contagious you know" from the other mums.'
>
> Meto

Actually, it's not highly contagious if a little care is taken, and there's no need to keep your child away from others, especially if it's possible to cover the ringworm with clothes or a dressing of some sort. Feel free to respond, therefore, with a patronising head tilt and a Mumsnetty 'Did you mean to be so rude?'; otherwise smile, nod and add them to your mental voodoo list of people you'll give a dose of threadworms to should a genie ever offer. And when they come whining to you about that, we suggest the following response:

'I had ringworm once. I can lend you my cow-bell if you like.'

EccentricaGallumbits

AMAZING RINGWORM FACT
As well as being able to catch ringworm from your pet you can actually give it to them, too, by stroking them with the infected area (though we're sure you can think of something more improving to do with a rainy Sunday afternoon).

Warts and Verrucas

(Why Oliver Cromwell's rule might have been easier with duct tape)

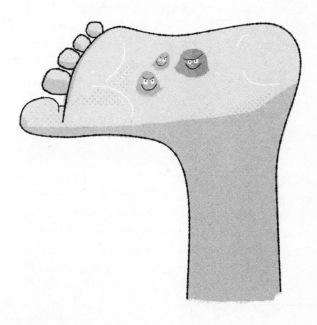

As Edwin Starr famously sang[*], 'Warts. (Huh. Yeah!) What are they good for? Absolutely NOTHING.' However, this doesn't mean that if your child picks one up, they aren't immense fun to try to get rid of.

KNOW YOUR ENEMY

WART (*verruca vulgaris*)
Warts are caused by the HPV (Human Papilloma Virus), which encourages the overproduction of the hard protein keratin in the epidermis. 'Common' warts appear on the fingers or hands and are small, oval, raised bumps, brownish in colour, with the appearance of cauliflower. A verruca is simply a wart on the foot.

STRENGTH: 3
Though harmless, warts are immune to most common disinfectants, so getting rid of them is tricky.

AGILITY: 0
Warts are spread through touch, but HPV isn't nearly as contagious as many viruses, so holding hands, for example, is unlikely to give your child a wart. They're more easily spread when the skin

[*]or may not have done.

is wet or damaged (hence swimming pools being a fecund breeding ground).

SKILLS: 4
Doing deals with the devil, magically transporting from one human to another via a white steed, killing toads. (Allegedly.)

SPEED: 0
In absolutely no hurry at all.

INTELLIGENCE: 3
One of the few viruses regularly seen off using witchcraft – a force to be reckoned with, cerebrally speaking.

ACHILLES HEEL
Many – including raw meat, urine and pounds sterling.

Warts we have known

Warts are not only the domain of witches. Some of this country's greatest and most good have worn a wart with pride. Oliver Cromwell had one, and is thought to be the originator of the expression 'warts and all'. It's said that after his death, the wart was removed and donated to the Society of Antiquaries, where it lived out its days visiting society dinner parties in a matchbox to 'amuse guests'. So if your child is getting a hard time because of a wart, you can tell them to inform their friends they are in good company.

Warding off warts; vanquishing verrucas

Really, the best course of action for warts and verrucas (unless painful or otherwise troublesome) is to leave them be and wait for them to go of their own accord. Frankly, however, we don't think 'just leaving it' is really in the spirit of this book, so we haven't let that stop us.

We'll assume, therefore, that you've tried either Bazuka or Wartner, or whatever mysterious alchemy Boots has on offer these days, and are ready to move on to more creative solutions. Here is a collection of cures ranging from the bizarre to the ridiculous. They may or may not work for your child, but they'll help to pass a rainy half-term if nothing else.

Saliva

A bit of spit and polish was good enough for your nan and it's also effective on a wart.

> 'When I was fourteen I had twenty-odd warts all on one hand. I read something that said you had to lick each wart first thing in the morning, before eating or drinking anything. Some enzymey thingy in saliva apparently contains antibodies. I did it for a week and within another ten days they had all gone.'
>
> Bucharest

Be warned, though, there is a danger you can spread said wart to your own tongue or lips this way, which is not a good look. If you'd rather not take the risk, we've good news: research by Mumsnetters has found dog saliva does the job, too.

> 'When I was little I had a few warts on my finger. My mum kept saying: "You'll have to get a dog to lick them." I thought she was mad, but then one day a dog did happen to lick my hand where the warts were. Gone in a week, I swear!'
>
> PuppyMonkey

If you don't own a dog and can't face explaining to a friend that you want their much-loved pet to lick away your child's warts, then perhaps simply roll the child in some Winalot Prime and pack them off to the park?

Amphibia

Legend has it that rubbing a toad on a wart makes it magically disappear (the wart, not the toad). This instruction varies slightly from country to country. The Spaniards believe you actually have to get the toad to bite the wart off, which may prove tricky. Another cure calls for you to rub the toad on the wart, then place the toad in a bag strung around your neck and wear it until the toad dies. We'd suggest you save that method until last.

Vegetation

A piece of banana peel taped to the offending growth has a good record of success. If keeping the peel stuck in the right place proves tricky, you can scrape a bit away from the inside of the skin and use it as a poultice on a plaster.

> 'It's a bit fiddly and you have to be patient – it took a month – but one morning we removed the banana skin and the verruca fell out, leaving a little hole, which then healed up.'
>
> Carolinecupcake

'The cure I've heard is to rub the wart with the inner skin from a broad bean.'

Chottie

Yes, the furry inside of a broad bean pod apparently has a similar effect. The wart is said to shrivel up and die after a few days. Got to be worth a shot before the toad, at least. And if your Abel & Cole box doesn't come up with the goods you need this week (it really is always kale and Jerusalem artichokes in those things, isn't it?) a humble dandelion may do just as nicely:

'My daughter had warts. The GP tried everything: cream, filing them. . . Then a friend of a friend said he had exactly the same thing. He told us to split the stalk of a dandelion and rub the juice all over the warts before bed and leave it to soak in. No word of a lie, within a week or so they were all gone.'

MossChops30

Other comestible cures

An ever-popular solution for all sorts of bugs and parasites, good old apple cider vinegar is worth a try, though you do run the risk of your child smelling like fish and chips, which is only mildly less excluding in a playground scenario than having a wart.

'Soak the pad of a plaster in cider vinegar and apply – keep doing so for a week. Maybe over half-term. . .'

Waswondering

Also stinky but effective is this:

'My podiatrist told me to try garlic oil on my three-year-old's verrucas. Getting the oil was a bugger. I crushed the garlic then squeezed the oil through a piece of muslin/net. But I put it on every night under a plaster and it worked! It stimulates the body's immune system, apparently.'

CanIBorrowSomeLuck

If you're a fan of a witchy solution, or something your nan might have sworn by, the steak method is fun:

'Rub your child's warts with a piece of steak then bury the steak in the garden. Within a month the warts will disappear. My mum used it on us in the 70s, before over-the-counter wart remedies were available and it always worked.'

Eekamoose

The 'theory' is that as the steak rots, so will the wart. We didn't say this was a cure rooted in science.

The Caveat Emptor method

> 'Just remembered I read (probably on Mums-net) about someone having a verruca and their grandad buying it off them. He gave them a coin and it went.'
>
> *Pogosticks*

Many still swear by the 'buy them off you' method for warts and verrucas. If you can't persuade a kindly stranger to buy your child's warts, you may have to offer to buy them yourself.

However, there is a similar method with an evil twist. Instead of persuading someone to buy the warts, you lumber an unsuspecting soul with them without telling them. Folklore says that if you see someone riding a white horse, you can touch your wart, look at the rider and say 'I wish you had my wart' to transfer it to them. Sneaky.

If you happen to live rurally, or in the nine-teenth century, you could try the following: rub an ear of corn on the offending growth, throw it out the door and the chicken who eats the corn will get your child's wart. Serves her right, too.

Death by Goth
Especially useful for verrucas, which need to be covered for swimming anyway, this method works

by starving them of fresh air and daylight. Cover the wart in black duct tape and keep it covered, removing occasionally to file it down a bit. It should start listening to My Chemical Romance and writing bad poetry in its bedroom before sloping off.

'I watched a TV programme recently where doctors did clinical testing on medical treatments that patients told them about. They tested duct-taping a verruca and had really positive results'.

Thants

'I painted my daughter's with black nail varnish to obscure the light. Gone after about ten days but needed topping up after baths while still there.'

Merlypussedoff

Absolute lunacy methods
Because we can't resist a cure for anything that begins: 'Give your child a dead cat and send them to a graveyard.'

'One of the most bizarre folk cures for warts involves taking a dead cat to a graveyard at midnight. As soon as you hear a noise, you're supposed to throw the cat in its general direction.

It was believed the sound came from the devil.
As the cat is thrown, the person throwing it
must say, "Cat follow the devil and warts follow
the cat.'"

FrannyandZooey

We would like to assure readers that no cats (or
devils) were harmed during the production of
this book.

'You need to walk widdershins around a yew
tree at midnight, naked and banging a saucepan.'

Greensleeves

If that doesn't get rid of them, then at least it will
give the neighbours something to talk about for
years to come.

AMAZING WART FACT
A wart was found on the mummified remains of
an Egyptian court musician, thought to be from
around 2400 BC. Your child's will almost certainly
clear up faster than that.

Molluscum

(How the war was won
with a toothpick)

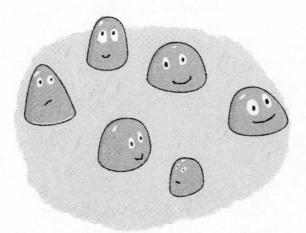

With its impressively bubonic appearance and a moniker that appears to have been lifted straight out of a Hogwarts spell book, moluscum contagiosum is the most medieval of childhood nasties. Its tendency to turn up without warning and hang around for months on end, meanwhile, calls to mind the sort of irritating house guest who promises to be gone in a few days, yet is still to be found languishing on your sofa three months later. But panic not: there are means of eviction. Read on to discover how to retain your composure in the face of an invasion, as well as a few tricks that might just help show it the door.

KNOW YOUR ENEMY

MOLLUSCUM (molluscum contagiosum)
A viral skin infection caused by the Poxviridae family (lovely couple; cute kids). Most common in children under six. Presents as small, reddish, dome-shaped spots with a yellowy-white 'core', in clusters on the trunk, limbs and sometimes face. Doesn't hurt, but can be itchy.

STRENGTH: 4
Their yellow core is like a tiny evil heart. Unchecked, they can hang about for years; badly

tackled, they can leave chicken pox-esque scars.
Not to be sniffed at.

AGILITY: 1

Pretty much static: tricky, but not impossible, to
pass on. Use a waterproof plaster before swimming, and avoid sharing towels, flannels or baths
with an infected person.

SKILLS: 3

Limited – but can live on the skin undetected by
the body's immune system for some time, which
is pretty impressive.

SPEED: 1

Slow – but that's its secret weapon. It spreads
slowly. . . and leaves slowly, too.

INTELLIGENCE: 1

Bottom set. But keen to learn.

ACHILLES HEEL

Cocktail sticks and dogged patience.

The official NHS recommendation is to leave molluscum to shuffle off of its own accord, as it's not actually harmful. However, it tends to spread around the body, and you may find clusters appearing for a couple of years: not a huge problem if they're on your child's legs, but potentially upsetting if they're on their face or somewhere equally visible. If you feel the need to take some sort of action, therefore, there are several things you can attempt to show the molluscum the door.

ROUTE ONE: GENTLE PERSUASION

The Bob Geldof method (Band Aid: geddit?)
Covering molluscum spots won't kill them, but it will help stop them from spreading, and may even irritate them enough to trigger an immune response (more of this later).

> 'I put those little Compeed plasters over them and it's worked a treat. They seem to die under there and dry up quickly after.'
>
> Minkersmum

> 'After years of the things, the doctor told us to put a plaster over each one. They were gone in three weeks. When they burst the spores

explode over the skin, creating new ones; by preventing the explosion they all die out. We were amazed!'

LeeCoakley

The Jamie Oliver method

As with most childhood nasties, molluscum is nothing a few middle-class ingredients can't solve. Mumsnetters variously recommend the application of apple cider vinegar, posh honey or olive oil. If they don't see off the spots, you can always make a marinade.

'Try Manuka honey. My two-year-old had spots for four months, and they were spreading. We applied it twice a day and within three weeks they were gone.'

Waterbabyabroad

The Holland and Barrett method

There are various herbal treatments, tinctures and essential oils you can try, either on the skin or in your child's bath. Don't forget that many essential oils will need to be diluted in carrier oil as they can burn the skin when used neat.

'I've recently started adding grapefruit seed extract and tea tree oil to my daughter's bath and putting the same diluted in olive oil directly onto the spots. They're now considerably smaller. The difference was noticeable within 48 hours.'

MrsAlwaysRight

'Try lemon myrtle oil, diluted in the bath (dissolving it in liquid soap first makes it easier). It stops the auto-inoculation. I got rid of my son's in six weeks.'

Shitmagnet

'We sent off for something called ZymaDerm – a tea-tree-based non-drug remedy. I'd recommend it to anyone.'

Happyrock

'Comfrey cream. It's the only thing that really works.'

Gooseberrybushes

The Eight Hour 'miracle' method

We've no idea why this works, but Elizabeth Arden Eight Hour Cream comes up time and again as a favourite cure. Worst-case scenario: it doesn't work but you've got yourself a very nice moisturiser. Either way, this method scores points for glamour, but loses them for, disappointingly, taking longer than eight hours to work.

'I got rid of my son's with it. May have been a fluke, but the spots went in less than two weeks.'

MadameCasatfiore

The inside-out method
The theory here is that you need to battle the enemy from within. Molluscum is a virus: strengthen your child's immune system, and he or she should be able to get rid of it more easily.

'My son had it for three years, slowly spreading over torso, back of knees and elbows. I'd always been advised to leave it alone, but when he began to get really upset, I felt he needed to see me try to help. I started him on oral probiotic drops (gut and immune system being best mates, you see). Three days later they started receding. Within two weeks … gone.'

Waltonswatcher1

ROUTE TWO: HARDCORE EVICTION
If you've not had success with the milder methods, now may be the time to get physical. Squeezing, popping or pricking molluscum spots is not recommended by healthcare professionals, as it can hurt, and you run the risk of scarring (physically

and possibly mentally, too, depending on how vigorous you are with your tweezers). That said, many parents do squeeze, and many report enormous success. If you try it, though, go gently, make *hygiene* your watchword – and don't tell anyone we told you to do it.

The theory goes that in order to fight off the molluscum virus the body's immune response needs to be triggered. Unsqueezed, the spots are self-contained, so your child's body is oblivious to them. By 'agitating' them (pricking or rubbing with a towel after a bath), you disturb the infectious centre and the body starts to fight them off.

> 'When I got a few I squeezed out the core and swabbed with alcohol and they never spread. The issue with kids is, it's hard to have a controlled squeezing because "patient compliance" is low.'
>
> *Charitycase*

Anything you can do to encourage the cores to the surface will make it easier to agitate or remove them, so try a hot bath or any natural product that might draw them out. Once the core is protruding, it's much easier to deal with.

'I treated my daughter's spots as I do verrucas: soaked cotton balls in apple cider vinegar and taped them on for a few hours each night. On the third night one had been bleeding; I squeezed it and the core came out.'

Stressedtothehilt

'My son had one big angry one on his chest. The core was protruding, so we gave him a hot bath, sterilised some tweezers and plucked. Gave it a gentle squeeze and the inside came easily. A few days later, all the others started protruding so we did the same. All disappeared within days.'

Winks123

Essentially, this sounds like a game of molluscum whack-a-mole, which does have a certain appeal. Remember though: it can be really painful. Do everything you can to numb the area first – and have a BIG bag of chocolate buttons to hand for afterwards.

'I bought some EMLA cream (local anaesthetic). My son didn't feel a thing, and I was squeezing and pressing hard with my nails.'

GordonPym

If you're too squeamish to squeeze, some parents have succeeded by just agitating the spots. This would seem to go against everything you know (when was the last time you gave a wasp a gentle slap, rather than the full weight of your sandal?) but in theory, it should work. Here's how to do it:

> 'Pierce a couple of the largest spots with a toothpick dipped in iodine. The spots react (go all red and angry-looking). This sets up a reaction and all the spots go red, then they all go! It took about a month from the piercing, but it was amazing. It's the trauma to the skin. The body recognises and then fights them. Or something. Anyway, it's one of the best things I've ever learned from Mumsnet.'
>
> Minicronperseiegg

> 'I had total success with the iodine and cocktail stick method. I got the information from an old dermatology book when I was a medical rep.'
>
> Alypaly

So, squeezing is controversial but we can't argue with the anecdotal evidence. In the end, it's up to you – a molluscumconundrum, if you will. And while we're looking at controversial cures. . .

ROUTE THREE: OFF THE BEATEN TRACK
It's not for everyone – but many Mumsnetters have reported success with homeopathy. If you're a fan, or even of the 'can't do any harm' persuasion, you might want to give it a go.

> 'My four-year-old had molluscum for a year and nothing worked. The pharmacist recommended Nelson's Thuja 6c tablets and within a fortnight it all cleared up. Very happy household – and far cheaper than the other treatments.'
>
> *Mrss79*

> 'I took my two-year-old to a homeopath on the advice of Mumsnetters. I was massively sceptical but he was too little to cope with squeezing, so I decided to give it a try. And I swear to God: it worked! After a consultation, she gave us two remedies to give that night. Next day all the spots came up red and inflamed, then just gradually disappeared over the next week. No scarring and no pain. I honestly didn't expect it would work but it genuinely appears to. I would definitely recommend it.'
>
> *Shergarandspies*

Whatever your chosen method, one thing's for sure: the meek may inherit the earth but it's the strong-stomached vizzigoths who cope best when molluscum strikes.

> 'My son had molluscum when he was eight. One day at school (I work there too) his teacher came running to tell me to stay calm, but that he had had quite a serious accident. She took me to the first aid room and whispered that he'd slipped on the rope bridge, caught his chest, and "sliced off his nipple". I lifted his T-shirt to discover he'd burst his molluscum. The look of horror on his teacher's face still makes me giggle.'
>
> Marymoocow

AMAZING MOLLUSCUM FACT

Molluscum can migrate to any part of the body, except the palms of hands and soles of feet.

Conjunctivitis

(Why your boobs need target practice)

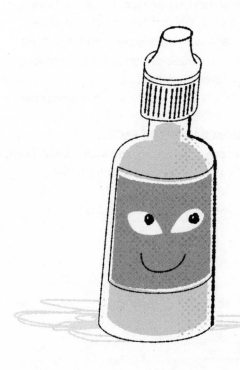

It's a parenting truth universally acknowledged that each of your child's orifices will at some point expel something unattractive, foul-smelling and likely to dry to a fine crust on your clothes. Eyes are no exception – and a gunged-up eye makes for a miserable child. So you need a few tricks up your sleeve to ease the symptoms as soon as they start.

KNOW YOUR ENEMY

EYE GUNGE (oculus 'orribilis)

Conjunctivitis comes in two 'brands': infectious (bacterial or viral) and allergic (non-infectious and caused by irritants such as smoke, dust, pollen or pet hair). It's a sticky customer, oozing in a range of shades, glueing eyelids together and causing bad tempers all round.

STRENGTH: 1

Poor. A quick trip to the pharmacist via the GP should sort it.

AGILITY: 3

May leap from one human to another, especially between children, since telling them not to rub their itchy eye is as likely to be effective as telling Kim Kardashian to stop taking selfies.

SKILLS: 2

Glues a child's entire face shut during sleep;
loiters on flannels and towels.

SPEED: 2

Takes hold quickly, but leaves with equal speed.

INTELLIGENCE: 2

Bottom set, generally speaking. A flexible
approach to infection but not stretching itself.

ACHILLES HEEL

Breast milk, medication, good hygiene.

Spotting signs of attack

A red and slightly swollen eye and your child's face looking like it's been stuck together with snot first thing in the morning are the killer signs; on the plus side, they're fairly hard to miss, so diagnosis tends to be speedy and decisive. The gunge is your key to identifying the species. Bacterial conjunctivitis is accompanied by an opaque yellow or greeny ooze and often arrives with the dog-end of a cold (after they've spent days religiously smearing snot into their eyes). The viral sort tends to be clearer, but sticky. If it's the allergic variety, you'll be looking at a clear, watery discharge. An allergic reaction usually occurs in both eyes simultaneously, while bacterial or viral conjunctivitis tends to start in one eye and then spread to the other.

You can clean the eyes very gently using cotton wool dipped in cooled, boiled water. Use a new piece of cotton wool for each eye to prevent cross-infection and wipe carefully from the inside corner of the eye to the outside one.

Very young babies are susceptible, having sometimes picked up bacteria in the birth canal. If yours has conjunctivitis before four weeks old, talk to your midwife or GP sooner rather than later as there can be complications at this age.

Getting shot of the gunge
Your GP can prescribe antibiotic eye drops for bacterial versions, drops that reduce the soreness for viral types, and an antihistamine if it seems to be an allergic reaction.

If your child has had conjunctivitis before, and you're sure you've identified it correctly, you can try tapping up a friendly pharmacist.

> 'You can get chloramphenicol over the counter for children over two. So I'd nip to the chemist rather than GP unless there are other concerns.'
>
> FestiveFreidaWhingesAgain

And once you've deftly applied the eye drops a few times and your child has blinked gratefully, everything should clear up nicely. The End.

We nearly had you there, didn't we?

How to get eye drops in
In reality, applying eye drops to a child is an experience more akin to attempting to shave a string bag full of cats while blindfolded. Babies are usually slightly more acquiescent, but for parents of toddlers and older children, here's how to ACTUALLY hit the target. . .

Pin them down. Firmly.

There are a few ways to handle this, depending on your offspring's size, strength and ability to pull a Houdini. If the child is reasonably compact, you can use the same method you would to get a pill into a cat: take a large bath towel, wrap them in it so only their head pokes out, get them in a rugby-ball hold under your arm and use the other hand to administer the drops.

'My best tip as a GP is that giving eye drops to a child is a two-person job. You can't do it by yourself! Babies you can – by tucking the head under your elbow. But a toddler is too big and wriggly.'

Neverenough

If the child is too large or agile, you'll need to use your weight against them:

'My technique, although it looked horrendous, was quite effective. I used to pin my daughter to the floor with my knees either side of her, so I was practically sitting on her (but not) then lean over her with my arms gripping her head, whilst at the same time trying to prise her eyes open. Tricky business but it did work.'

Lazylou

A couple of words of caution, at this point. Obviously don't *actually* put your weight on the child, and don't be tempted to use both hands to pin them down and squeeze the drops out by holding the bottle in your teeth. That way madness lies. Secondly, do go easy on the 'prising' of eyelids. In fact, there's a nifty way to avoid having to do this at all:

> 'My GP said to put the drops into the little well, at the corner of the eye, when the eye is shut, then when they open their eyes it will run in.'
>
> *Piratecat*

The method does assume that the child will willingly open their eyes at some point but, as long as you can prevent them turning their head or wiping their eyes until they've done so, you're home and dry. And for any stubborn little blighters who refuse to open their peepers, you can exclaim loudly 'Good lord! Look at that! The free ice cream van is here!' Infallible.

Bribe your child. . .
Now is not the time for high principles; nor is it the time for nutrition. Bin the raisins and dried banana and go straight for the big guns: chocolate

buttons or Haribo is what's going to get them through this, nothing less.

> 'We rewarded our son, age two, with Chocolate Buttons, one per eye. He now actually asks me for "Eyes, Mummy", knowing that he gets Buttons after. If I mention "eyes" he will lie on the floor and squint at me in preparation. Handy, as he has now had conjunctivitis three times this year.'
>
> Bonzo77

On top of choccies, adding a little luxury to the experience will help. A cushion for their head and anything else that makes it more comfortable is worth a shot.

> 'Eye drops are more tolerable when warm. Put the bottle in your front trouser pocket for twenty minutes before you dose so the liquid is almost at body temperature.'
>
> PrettyCandles

. . . or just bribe your GP

There are antibiotic preparations that don't actually require 'dropping' into the eye – so if you're having real trouble, try grovelling for something else.

'My DS (nearly three) HATED eye drops. The
GP prescribed antibiotic eye gel which he tol-
erated much better.'

Casserole

Other ways to fight the ooze
If you can't get to a GP immediately, or think
you've only got a mild case on your hands, there
are a few alternative remedies that can help clear
up an eye infection such as conjunctivitis. A very
mild salt solution acts as an antiseptic and helps
with healing (but don't make it too strong as it
can sting). Here are a few other mild solutions that
might help:

Tea and sympathy

Pop a tea bag into a clean mug, pour boiling water
on, whip the teabag out and leave the water to
cool. You can then dip cotton wool into it and gently bathe the affected area. It seems to help soothe
and relieve itching – and there's something pleas-
ingly 'blitz spirit' about popping on the kettle to
deal with a health issue, too.

'Cold tea is even better than salt water, as
the tannins act as anti-inflammatories. Old-
fashioned, but works.'

Lonecatwithkitten

Certain herbal teas have the same effect.

> 'A doctor recommended a camomile tea solution and it was the dog's bollocks at getting rid of eye gunk.'
>
> BNMum

If your child is allergic to flowers such as asters and chrysanthemums, however, give this one a miss as it can cause a reaction. Stick with the PG Tips.

No more tears
For reasons unknown, a weak solution of Johnson's Baby shampoo seems to have cleared up a gungy eye for many a Mumsnetter. It's widely recommended for the symptoms of blepharitis, and some GPs recommend it for a mild case of viral conjunctivitis. While it's not a miracle cure, it may help clean the area gently, particularly if your child is waking with their eyes glued shut each morning and if cooled, boiled water isn't doing the trick.

> 'My GP recommended a weak solution of Johnson's Baby – worked a treat.'
>
> SirChenJin

Miracle mammaries

For a solution that's as natural as they come, nothing beats a squirt of breast milk – though obviously you'll need to be breastfeeding for this one to work.

But wait! Before you whip off your bra, a word of caution. Give the child fair warning first. There *are* people who enjoy being chased by women waving their breasts and squirting milk at them, but that's a *very* niche adult market.

In terms of practicalities, you're unlikely to make a direct hit straight from the nipple so you'd be well advised to express first and use cotton wool or a syringe to administer it.

> 'If trying the breast-milk thing, express into a cup or similar and drop into the eye with a syringe – I couldn't squirt from my boob, my aim was well off!'
>
> *FloweryBoots*

Furthermore, there are other environmental hazards to consider:

> 'Husband held daughter on his lap while I tried to aim straight. Needless to say, he and I collapsed in fits of giggles and daughter ended up with milk EVERYWHERE (except

in her eye). Also remember to close the cur-
tains. I forgot.'

Squiggers

And if you really must, you can have a go on
yourself.

'I decided before I put it in his eye, I would try it
in my own just to make sure that it didn't sting.
I forgot I had my contact lenses in. . .'

Mawbroon

Still. . . impressive results to be had with 'an eyeful
for an eye', as recommended by the Good Book
itself. Goes to show that, as is so often the case, the
solution you've been searching for is right under
your nose. Literally.

AMAZING EYE FACT
There is no medical name for the gunge which
eyes occasionally emit during sleep. Sleepy dust,
eye bogies. . . you can officially call 'em whatever
you like.

Foreign Objects

(Why what goes up must come down)

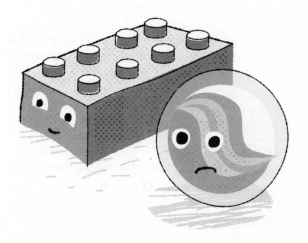

Why do children feel the need to insert things into orifices? As George Mallory said of Everest: because they're there.

KNOW YOUR ENEMY

FOREIGN OBJECT (*alienum objectum*)

From marbles to Maltesers, any item small enough is fair game. Insertion of foreign objects is most common in children aged between six months and four years.

STRENGTH: 4

This is not a nasty to take on alone. Take your child to A&E and let a professional go into battle.

AGILITY: 4

Impressive. You wouldn't think it possible to swallow a Lego brick, would you? Or cram a whole Cheerio up a nostril? Think again.

SKILLS: 4

Points for rage-induction. Invisibility on being swallowed (no matter how meticulously you rake through poo for the Micro Machine wheel, it'll be a miracle if you ever see it again).

SPEED: 4
Turn your back for a second and that sweetcorn
will be straight down the ear canal.

INTELLIGENCE: 2
Not big and NOT clever. <hard stare>

ACHILLES HEEL
Common sense. And tweezers.

Welcome to parenthood. Please leave your nerves at the door.
If you aren't already familiar with that stomach-through-floor moment when you ask 'You stuck it WHERE?', rest assured that it's a matter of when, not if. Here's how it'll go down:

1. The incident will occur on a Friday between the hour the surgery closes and your second glass of wine (just big enough to mean a taxi is your only option).
2. Not having *seen* them stick the object into the orifice in question, you'll retain a nagging doubt as to whether they made the whole thing up and you're sitting in A&E for four hours for nothing.
3. Having been through the horror of hospital trip, removal and a thorough telling-off, they will promptly do it again.

There are two types of Foreign Object Incident: things that work their way *through* (items swallowed) and things that need to come out the way they went in (primarily noses and ears; occasionally bottoms). We did hear once of an unfortunate mother who had to take her toddler to A&E with a marble stuck under his foreskin. The mind boggles.

Down the hatch

If you think the object might be dangerous, or if your child is very young, they need to see a doctor. There are a few items for which you need to rush them to hospital (button batteries, poisons such as slug pellets, anything corrosive – such as dishwasher tablets – or anything sharp), but whatever they've swallowed, look out for ill effects (problems breathing, eating or drinking; blueish tinges around the mouth; pain in the chest or stomach; dribbling or vomiting). If you have ANY concerns, whip them into A&E.

In general, though, if the item is smallish, smoothish and non-toxic, you don't need to go to DEFCON 1 immediately. Plastic items such as Lego (henceforth known as 'bloody Lego') won't show up on an X-ray, so as long as it hasn't got stuck, the doctor will probably tell you to go home and wait it out.

When a doctor says 'wait it out', what they mean is 'wait until they poo it out' (should bloody Lego be the culprit, the correct medical term is, of course, 'shitting a brick'). Usually, this takes a couple of days but it can be as many as ten. It's not advisable to give laxatives, but a bit of roughage will do no harm.

'When my sister swallowed a tiny key, the doctor told my mum to feed her porridge to coat any sharp edges and it passed through without a problem.'

Suedonim

As ever, where children are concerned, things can always get worse. Steel yourself for the day they move on from Lego to more, errm, *animate* fare. It may be less dangerous (it is, after all, organic) but it's likely to be far, far more disgusting.

'My son, aged three, ate a spider – one of those huge ones. I saw three legs on his chin, but even the thought of my child eating a spider didn't make me brave enough to retrieve it. I gave him water and hoped he'd swallow, which he did. He eventually went on to eat a few woodlice and a worm.'

Insanityscatching

'My daughter, at 14 months, ate a spider's nest… If they'd come out of her nappy she'd have been going to live with her grandparents.'

YouBastardSockBalls

Other orifices
Children, like nature, abhor a vacuum. Give them a tiny toy and chances are they'll stick it somewhere. Items in nostrils, ears, bottoms and anywhere

similar do usually need medical attention – it's very easy to make the situation worse yourself.

Smells like toddler spirit

Noses are a popular target. If the first you know of the object's existence is the moment it emerges again, don't feel bad; you'll by no means be the first parent to have had no idea their kid was wandering around with a contraband item up their hooter.

> 'I know of a child who started to smell awful and no one could work out why. Turned out she'd shoved a Barbie's shoe up her nose and infection had set in. The visit to A&E was pretty gruesome.'
>
> *NippieSweetie*

Advice differs on whether or not low-key interventions are possible. But it's worth encouraging the child to blow their nose to see if that shifts it:

> 'My son did this with an inch-long piece of cooked macaroni. He snorted it out by holding one nostril shut and blowing through the other. It was like that magician trick where they pull a string of flags from their hand!'
>
> *Soupdragon*

Do try to keep older siblings, whose 'help' may not be welcome, well out of the incident area, however.

> 'My daughter shoved a popcorn kernel up her nose. Had almost got her to blow it out when her elder sister said, "Yes, like this." SNIFF... We went to A&E to get it suctioned.'
>
> SurprisedJerseySpud

Many swear by the 'parents' kiss' method of removal – in fact, some doctors do, too, but opinion on whether it's OK to attempt this at home varies, so exercise caution:

> 'Close your child's other nostril, seal your mouth over his mouth and give a short, sharp blow. This pushes air up the back of the nose and forces the object out.'
>
> Porpoise

Think that's impressive? Props, then, for the parents whose ingenuity in the face of a foreign object leaves the rest of us standing:

> 'My son got a magnetic ball stuck up his nostril. My husband, in a breathtaking moment of inspiration, got it out with another magnet!'
>
> Hassled

But if a lucky sneeze or a partner with masses of initiative is not forthcoming, you'll be making your way to A&E. While it's not common, it is possible for items up the nose to be aspirated into the lungs, so while this one isn't an ambulance call, you do need to get them there as soon as you can.

On a positive note, the more ridiculous the item, the more certain you can be that your child will be the talk of medics' dinner parties up and down the country the following weekend ('He stuck a WHAT up there?' 'Yes, I KNOW! I didn't even think Playmobil DID toilet brushes. . .'). Here are a few tales of nasal woe from mums whose kids will have surely made the A&E hall of fame.

> 'Nephew got a Lego man's head stuck up his nose. It was looking down at the doctor when he looked up his nostril.'
>
> *Charlie97*

> 'My daughter shoved a tiny screw in her nostril. We went to A&E where they got it out and she wanted to keep it. So we did. Then, SHE SHOVED IT BACK UP THERE. So back we went.'
>
> *Nobodyliveshere*

'Mine did this with a piece of plastic wrapping. We went to the doctor, me saying, "No way would she put something up her nose and not tell me." Out came a piece of plastic covered in green slime…"I didn't tell you Mummy because I thought you'd be cross."'

Jacanne

Cheers, big ears

If you've got an ear situation, get the child in question to tip their head so the ear with the object in it is pointing to the floor. In this position, gently pull the ear slightly out and back, which can sometimes straighten the ear canal and the object may drop out. If not, get to A&E. Don't be tempted to try tweezers yourself. The chance of them suddenly turning their head, causing you to force the object further in, is too great.

If they haven't told you they've done it, you might notice their hearing deteriorates, or that they're complaining of noise in their ear. Food items get smelly quickly, so if your child has an unusual aroma about them (a sort of eau de rotting dead goat) it's worth asking a few questions.

'When my daughter was in hospital, we met a boy who was there to have grommets fitted as his hearing had become almost non-existent.

He returned from the operating theatre with a small tube of gravel and perfect hearing.'

Marriednotdead

Doctors are virtually unshockable. They will have removed all manner of unmentionables from all manner of folks. Your child's Playmobil-in-the-ear pales into insignificance. Usually. . .

'When my eldest was three and getting deafer and deafer in one ear I took him to the GP thinking "ear wax". Nope. The little horror sat in the GP's office and confessed to putting his bogies in there.'

QueenRollo

And if you're currently reading this from a sweaty, plastic chair in A&E, with your child beside you, marble up nose, and wondering which animal sacrifice you failed to make in a previous life. . . Well, you could be the mum of this child:

'A three-year-old I had dealings with was found to have seventeen cherry pips up her vagina. She thought it was a tidy way to dispose of them. They did all come out. Eventually.'

PacificDogwood

There's always someone worse off than yourself, isn't there?

AMAZING FOREIGN OBJECT FACT

Research from the University Hospital of Wales on how quickly sweets dissolved inside the nose found that Smarties took 30 to 35 minutes to dissolve, while Polos took a whopping 45 to 50 minutes. TicTacs took just 20 to 25 minutes.

Vomit

(Why not everything is
'better out than in')

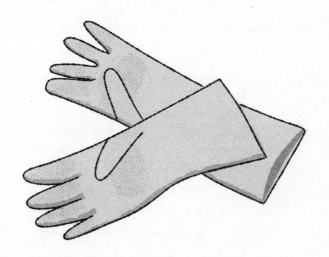

Nature breaks you in gently where puke is concerned. On becoming a parent, you get several months of tiny milky sick-ups to practise on. Possets (so tame they named them after a pudding) are blobs of curdled milk, silently expelled onto your shoulder; you will at some point find you have been round Waitrose, met friends for lunch and done the school run with one on your lapel. As kids get older, however, milky-scented possets become voluminous oceans of noxious fluid that charge from your child, enveloping everything in their wake, 1950s-B-movie style. The good news is there are plenty of ways to see it off your carpet, sofa, clothes and duvets. Marigolds at the ready: we're going in.

KNOW YOUR ENEMY

VOMIT (*emesis revoltimus*)
There are examples of vomiting in art from 500 BC, and vomiting looms large in our modern-day collective consciousness, from Monty Python's Mr Creosote to little Regan with her 'boundary-testing' behaviour in *The Exorcist*.

STRENGTH: 3
Certainly smells strong. Has the ability to adhere tenaciously to textured surfaces, such as sofas.

AGILITY: 4

A good projectile vomit can cover a surprising amount of ground.

SKILLS: 4

Its viscous nature allows it to slip out of the tiniest hole in a plastic carrier bag, yet turn instantly to concrete on impact with any surface.

SPEED: 3

Varies, but it's between 10mph and 20mph.

INTELLIGENCE: 2

More creative than academic.

ACHILLES HEEL

Bicarbonate of soda.

Preventing the advances of puke
Vomit may have the element of surprise, but you
have the razor-sharp prepping skills that come
with parenthood. If you suspect a puke is immi-
nent, shore up your trenches pre-bedtime with a
bed that is battle-ready. Invest in a second waterproof mattress protector, and make the bed up
with two sheets and two mattress protectors so
that after a puke you can simply whip off the top
layers and change the duvet cover. Some canny
parents leave the bed permanently made up like
this – saves on airing cupboard space, too. You can
always substitute the second mattress protector for
a towel.

> 'My son's bed is always made up in double.
> When he's sick it's easy to take the top layer off
> and carry on with the night.'
>
> *Ispidermanyoumeanpirate*

Here are a few more neat tricks for Amber Vomit
Alert days:

> 'I spread a large bath towel on the floor so he
> can be whipped out of bed and placed on the
> towel to catch most of it.'
>
> *Harlettoscara*

'As well as towels, I put cheap IKEA fleece blankets down. Fleece is water-resistant, so the vomit doesn't soak in.'

Velmadinkley

'Puppy mats are my tip. Very cheap from pound shops. Put on the floor below bed or sofa in case of over-edge spewing.'

Gastonschesthair

In terms of receptacles, there are a plethora from which to take your pick. The trusty retired washing-up bowl is always a sensible option; on the other hand, one enterprising Mumsnetter said she was the proud owner of a 'sick wok'. By all means, if you've a surfeit of woks, do the same. If not, here are some more prosaic ways to catch puke.

'A potty is good if your child finds a proper bucket too big on their lap.'

Gruber

'Collect ice-cream tubs. Once you get a decent stash they can be binned after a couple of vomits.'

Godsavethequeen

Claiming your child back from desiccation

As with diarrhoea, children (particularly babies) can quickly become dehydrated, which is a big deal when you're tiny, so it's something you need to make a priority. Yes, even ahead of scraping vomit off the carpet.

Babies six months or under should just be given their normal milk, so if you're breastfeeding, continue to do so. Getting a few extra feeds in to keep their fluid levels up is also a good idea so offer a feed as often as you can. Perhaps have a good pile of muslins to hand, however. Breastfeeding a vomiting child is something of an extreme sport.

If you're concerned about dehydration with your baby, ask your GP or pharmacist about baby oral rehydration solutions or offering extra cooled, boiled water.

With older children, while it's fine for them not to eat for a day or so, it definitely isn't fine not to drink. Give them plenty of clear fluids – clear broth or just plain water (no fizzy drinks or fruit juice until they're a bit better). When they start complaining about the Dickensian nature of the menu you'll know they're on the mend. Oral rehydration solutions are great for replacing lost salts and electrolytes, too. If they aren't keeping anything down at all and you're concerned about dehydration, get them seen by a doctor.

And once they're on the road to recovery, pour yourself a stiff drink. You'll be in need of some fluids to build up your strength again yourself after all that.

Regurgitation detoxification
Finding yourself gingerly sniffing a cushion cover days after the vomiting has ceased? Here's how to rid your home of stains and nasty niffs.

Carpets and rugs
If you have only one carpeted room in your entire house, you can be sure your vomiting child will gravitate to it like an 80%-wool-20%-nylon-seeking missile. Particularly if it's cream. And especially if their last meal was tomato-based.

> 'Two mugs of water, one tablespoon each of white vinegar and handwash laundry detergent. Sponge over the stain and blot. Sponge over cold water to remove the solution.'
>
> *Moominsarehippos*

> 'We use 1001 Carpet Spray. It works a dream – gets rid of stains and smell.'
>
> *Ghosty*

Ah yes: the smell. Like Parmesan from Satan's own armpit. One tiny unnoticed splash can render the entire downstairs of a family home unliveable.

'Try bicarb. Make a weak solution with water, rub it in, let it dry, vac it out.'

JanH

'Give Zoflora a go. It's a concentrated disinfectant – took the smell of vom from the carpet and sofa right out!'

Saesometimes1

'Get one of the pet odour neutralisers that contain enzymes.'

Seona1973

While we're here, a quick word about sisal flooring. Well, three words: Never. Get. It. All that texture and rustic charm may look smart on the pages of Elle Decoration, but once you've had to clean vomit out of all those crevices, you'll be ready to rip it up and replace it with a nice, smooth, cheap sheet of lino.

'Sick on sisal flooring? You need lots of water (then lots of rubbing with a towel afterwards), a

soft-ish brush and lots of patience. I had to scrape
it out of all the carved-out bits with a butter knife.'

Ladyoftheflowers

Hard floors

An excellent choice: well done, you. However,
vomit travels fast on hard floors so a metric hell-
tonne of kitchen towel is required to stem the
flow. Sawdust is helpful. If you have none, try this:

'I use clumping cat litter for puddles on hard
surfaces, makes it less unpleasant to clean up.'

Wigglybeezer

Sofas

If your child has it in for you, they may sick up
on your sofa. Enjoy getting chunks of spew out
from the cushion piping with a cocktail stick.
Clean using whatever method your manufacturer
recommends. The truly prepared will have paid
for insurance so they send out a nice cleaning
operative to pick out the chunks with their own
proprietary cocktail stick. If all that's done and
the sofa still retains a stench of death, try this:

'On an inconspicuous place try shaving cream
(traditional bog-standard stuff not fancy gel). It's
great on sick smell.'

Pineapplebed

'Put some ground coffee in some tights and hang it in the room. The coffee absorbs the smell.'

Orangehead

Sheets, duvets and mattresses

There's something very visceral about being woken to rivers of vomit in the middle of the night. Remain calm if possible. In the immediate aftermath, if logistics allow, try to get the duvet cover outside and then follow these instructions:

'Hang it over a plastic chair and hose down. Then soak overnight with baking soda and vinegar in water. In the morning, bung it in the washing machine.'

Hairyhandedtrucker

If outside is not an option, take it to the bathroom and shower it in the tub. Hoick out anything (whole pieces of penne, for example) that might cause a plumbing issue and chuck something vicious down the plughole after it.

'I shower bedding first (cold so as not to set it) to get the chunks off. Then hot wash (if all cotton) with bio powder and a scoop of Vanish powder.'

DomesticSlattern

Once bedding and any collateral-damage cuddly toys are dealt with, turn your attention to the mattress.

> 'Use towels to soak up as much as you can. Spray a solution of biological washing powder onto the area and blot with more towels. Standing on the towel will help soak up moisture. Sprinkle baking soda over, leave overnight and vacuum off in the morning.'
>
> *Macdog*

If there's no option but to put the mattress back on the bed, clean it and turn it then give it an airing and deal with the smell the following day.

Public-place pukes

If there's one thing worse than an episode of vomiting, it's an episode in a public place. But there is one major upside: it wasn't on your carpet! In fact, if you're lucky you can chuck a bucket of water at it, or sand on it, and the whole thing is dealt with almost effortlessly.

> 'My son (age three) was suddenly and spectacularly sick in a shopping-centre car park. One of those men in blazers and earpieces walked past and offered to clean it up. Son was still a bit

upset so I slunk off. Later that week I sent a note thanking them. Imagine my surprise when by return of post I got a very effusive letter thanking me for thanking them (huh?) and enclosing a free top-of-the-range car valet token. May I suggest anyone wanting a free car-clean takes a manky-looking child to a shopping-centre car park pronto.'

Anchovy

The most fascinating thing about your child vomiting in public (bear with us) is the chance to study the parental reflex we call 'The Pietersen Puke Catch'. Spot your child on the brink of a public chunder and you will find yourself running towards them, palms cupped, ready to catch it.

If you're standing in an antique Chinese rug store in Knightsbridge, this reflex is handy. If not, you're doing yourself few favours. Firstly, your hands will never contain it all, so you'll end up like a stone cherub in a water feature, with a fountain of vomit trickling gently over the edge of your palms. Secondly, once caught, you have no spare hand with which to open a door or lift a loo seat to dispose of the vomit.

If you have the presence of mind, go for a receptacle that is not attached to your body. A plastic bag is good, provided you can empty your shopping out quick enough, but anything will do in an emergency.

'My little girl once threw up a bowl of spaghetti Bolognese while we were walking home. I automatically held her close to me. When we got home, I removed all our clothes, including my bra, which was basically two bags full of vomit. I did wonder whether that sort of thing ever happened to Madonna.'

Morningpaper

'A good solution in a tight spot (motorway; travel-sick nephew) was a clean nappy.'

Marriednotdead

'There was one epic time when I managed to catch it in his toy truck.'

Lola88

'My eldest vomited in my mouth when he was a baby. I was in WH Smith's. I swallowed it in front of a horrified queue.'

Pagwatch

There's certainly truth in the saying 'what doesn't kill you makes you stronger'. Now sip this water, have a lovely big sleep and you'll soon feel better.

AMAZING VOMIT FACT
The record for the longest distance covered by a projectile vomit is 27 feet.

Poo

(Counselling for the scatologically scarred)

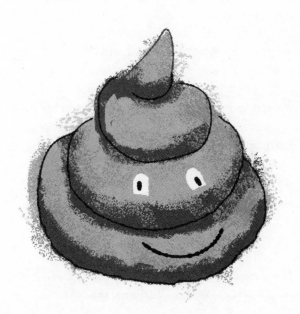

Shit happens – and if you're a parent-to-be, dealing with it is soon to become one of your primary duties. You're probably hoping that, while you're no big fan of faeces, when it comes to that of your precious infant, you'll feel differently. You won't. It may be your child's poo, but that doesn't change the fact that it is still, in essence, poo.

However, if you can familiarise yourself with the stuff at every age and stage, you'll at least be prepared for the onslaught. And while this may sound like cold comfort now, when you're confronted with your first up-the-back-and-out-the neck explosion, you'll thank us.

KNOW YOUR ENEMY

POO (*merdus abominatus*)
As old as humankind (the oldest poo ever discovered dates back 50,000 years), poo is as intrinsic a part of parenthood as sleepless nights and stepping on Lego. When it behaves itself, it's merely an unpleasant fact of life. At its most powerful, however, it can reduce grown men and women to tears.

STRENGTH: 4
The stench of a poo that's gone rogue can blind a wolf at thirty paces.

AGILITY: 3
Good on the whole; in fact it can, on occasion,
run wild. Sometimes, however, it lacks motivation
and gets stuck: in bowels, in toilet bowls, on
carpets. . .

SKILLS: 4
Has the devastating ability to adhere like glue
to virtually any surface (except, of course, that
of a shovel).

SPEED: 3
Very much dependent on consistency.

INTELLIGENCE: 2
Studies into the intelligence of poo itself are few,
but there's a recognised link between the scent
of a bookshop and needing to go; apparently
the smell of ink on paper stimulates the bowel.
Parents of early readers, beware.

ACHILLES HEEL
Soda crystals.

'It's just milk until they're on solids,' people will tell you, as you gag and heave while cleaning poo from every crevice. It's not 'just milk' though, is it? Let's be honest: it's crap. Crap that has less of the stench of death about it than that of a weaned child, but crap nonetheless. What's more, newborn-crap possesses the uncanny ability to get *everywhere*. Fail to change a full nappy at your peril: one good roll, and the contents will be up your infant's back like a greased weasel. But if you're slow off the blocks and expulsion occurs, here's how to cope.

Dealing with a 'poonami'

> 'Wait until your baby not only shits up the back and out the side of the nappy, but does so while you're out of the room and spreads the surplus crap all over the cream rug, white sofa, and their own FACE. That, reader, is a poonami.'
>
> Thefantasticfixit

Poonamis come in many shapes and sizes, from those that run silently out of both leg-holes and into your lap, to guerrilla versions that lie in wait until you have the nappy off in a public place.

> 'One that sticks in my memory is a change I did on the loo floor of a restaurant. The never-ending

poo that started the second I removed the nappy nearly finished me. It was like a malfunctioning Mr Whippy.'

Query Query

When disaster strikes, your focus must be on minimising collateral damage. The only thing you *have* to get clean is the baby; the order of things to save next should be based strictly on expense. And if you only ever remember one piece of parenting advice, let it be this: that envelope neck on a babygrow is there to save you from defecation devastation. Simply slide the babygrow down over their shoulders rather than up over the head, and you'll at least keep things contained.

If the poonami has completely taken out a babygrow, there are tips for resuscitation at the end of the chapter. If there's just no rescuing their clothes, though, don't look back. Ditch the outfit and save yourselves. Like we said: collateral damage.

Why intervention is never the answer
The most demoralising poo incidents are those in which we act as the architects of our own misery. Why, for the love of gravy, do we all at some point stick our fingers into a baby's nappy 'to check'? What do we *expect* to find in there? Banknotes?

'I once went in for a sniff and ended up with poo on my nose because the nappy was full to the brim.'

Soupdragon

On other occasions, nappies seem to work in league with our own stupidity:

'I thought I was being clever by pinching the side of the nappy with my thumb and forefinger, but it created a gaping hole from which the (runny, breastfed) poo slid into my lap.'

Essie3

The key to a happy relationship with nappies is as little interference as possible – and that goes for your child as well as for you. Despite waking you every two hours for a year, your child will manage one day to wake without crying, silently remove their nappy and smear the contents all over themselves, their bedding, their cot and anything else within reach. You'd think being hosed off in the shower at 2am would act as a deterrent, but inexplicably, once they've managed it, they tend to repeat the exercise. Here are a few tricks to try if you've got a dirty protester on your hands:

'Put their sleeping bag on back to front (i.e. zip at the back) and secure the zip with a nappy pin.'

Frogs

'Put babygrows on backwards so they can't undo them.'

Mum2girls

'Gaffer tape. Wrap it round the top of the nappy so they can't undo the tabs.'

Norem

Diarrhoea: just run with it

Let's be clear: there's a difference between diarrhoea and the frequently oozy contents of milk-fed babies' nappies. These tend to be less firm than the productions of those of the food-eating population, so if your newborn's poo is more liquid than solid, don't panic. If your weaned baby's nappies are still a little. . . *relaxed*, have a think about their diet. Fruit juice, for example, can go through them like a dose of salts, while other foodstuffs (eggs; bananas) might have the effect of firming things up.

If your child has the actual squits, however, tactics must be deployed. While in nappies diarrhoea is awful, but can at least be contained; it's once they're potty-trained that you'll truly learn to fear it. The worst-case scenario is that they come down with a tummy bug during potty training. If this should happen, try letting them wear pull-ups for a day or two. It might 'set them back' a bit, but frankly, crappy pants several times a day aren't going to fill them with confidence either, so you may as well do yourself and your carpet a favour. Older children are likely to be embarrassed by the thought of a nappy, so dig out the old pants, pop towels on much-loved items of furniture and cross your fingers.

Stomach bugs usually blow through in a couple of days, but if you want to hasten their departure, the following tricks are worth a try:

'Keep them off everything except dry bread/ plain biscuits and water for a day – usually allows the gut enough time to pass whatever it is and settle down.'

Thumbwitch

'Stewed apples are ideal binding food when recovering from a viral tummy upset.'

Whomovedmychocolate

The key thing, though, is to keep them hydrated. If your child shows signs of dehydration (dark or infrequent urine, no tears when crying, dizziness, dry mouth, skin that feels unusually cool) see a doctor. Beyond rehydration, recommendations are that children eat more or less normally as soon as they feel able. And that you keep the Carpet Doctor close to hand.

Constipation: let it flow
For older children, there are plenty of products available to get things moving, so a trip to Boots should do the trick if upping their water and fibre (dried apricots can work wonders) hasn't helped. It's with pre-weaned babies that things get trickier. Babies can go a truly awe-inspiring amount of time without a bowel movement, so the first thing to remember is that there's no need for panic, so long as they're still weeing. If they seem uncomfortable, though, there are lots of natural remedies you can try – but make sure you're on amber alert at all times for when it finally makes landfall.

'Do a cycling motion with their legs. And DUCK.'
Longdistance

'Google "reflexology for constipated babies". My daughter was quite constipated as a tiny baby, and the midwife showed me how to do it.'
Poledra

> 'Massage your baby's tummy, outwards in circles in a clockwise direction. Some oil or cream on your fingers can help.'
>
> *Nobodysfool*

After the event: clean-up techniques

If you thought getting poo out of your child's *body* was hard work, wait till it gets on your carpet. Assuming the strike is not so devastating that you must simply seal the room and burn everything within it, there are a few tricks that will help you recover.

Clothes

Due to their position on the front line, babygrows and vests take a helluva beating but even they can be brought back from the brink of death.

> 'Soak the item in some water with a Milton sterilising tablet.'
>
> *PebbleJones*

> 'Try Fairy liquid neat on the stain and then wash as normal. It must be the original green one – none other worked for me.'
>
> *Ilovegracieboo11*

And if you're daft enough to enter the scene without careful consideration for where you're putting your feet, here's how to get poo out of the treads of your shoes:

'Freeze the shoes overnight to make it easier to pick out the poo. If they're trainers, wash in the machine with Dettol afterwards.'

Vajazzler

Carpets

Dealing with a crappy carpet is true black-ops parenting stuff. Remove as much 'matter' as possible with baby wipes, then try any or all of the following store-cupboard solutions:

'Soda crystals. Make a solution, scrub it in, then use a steam cleaner on it.'

Brimfull

'Make a foam from washing-up liquid and work it in, follow with clear water, then put towels down and jump on them to dry the area.'

Sonilaa

'Flood with water and blot with loads of kitchen roll. Then use water with liquid detergent. Blot again. Then a teaspoon of ammonia in lots of water. Blot. Then plain water. Blot.'

Enid

'Vanish Powershot works a treat.'

Carrieboo

'Shaw's Stain and Soil Remover. Fantastic.'

Chandra

And if you're at the point of no return, there is a final solution:

'We moved house. Expensive, but it worked!'

Soupdragon

AMAZING POO FACT
Did you know there are four bags of astronaut poo still on the moon from when Neil Armstrong visited?

Dragons under the Bed

(And other witches, wolves and wild things)

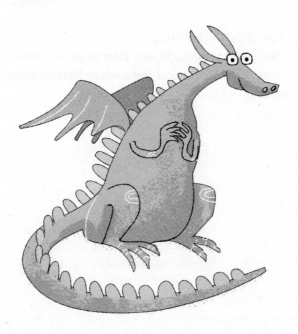

When a knight won his spurs in the stories of old, he was 'gentle and brave, gallant and bold'. If you're less 'gentle and brave' than 'knackered and tetchy', dig deeper. When it comes to dragons under the bed, monsters in the wardrobe and beasts lurking on the stairs, you are Queen's Champion for your child.

Being woken suddenly to deal with a witch, or even a walrus (more of that later), may test your patience, but even in the dark at 2am, there's nothing like the wide-eyed trust of a sleepy, sweaty-haired bairn to make you think, 'Damn it, I will slay that beast and the spaceship he rode in on. And I will PUT THAT BASTARD IN THE BIN.'

Read on for more ingenious and inventive ways to rid your home of every beastie and bogeyman, witch and warlock in (non-)existence.

KNOW YOUR ENEMY

UNDER-THE-BED BEASTIES (*monstra sub lecto*)
Parenting really stretches your CV. Thought having children wouldn't require you to slay anything more dastardly than a spider? Think again. The witches, tigers, monsters and more that you'll see off are as big, dark and wide-ranging as your child's imagination.

STRENGTH: 2

On paper, these guys have it all: big teeth, sharp claws and magic. But scratch the surface and they're pretty soft underneath.

AGILITY: 3

Varies. Dragons are good in the air, less so on the ground. Indeed, most monsters tend to be lumbering sorts. If dealing with a tiger or similar, you need to be pretty light on your feet.

SKILLS: 4

Dependent on species. May include flying, magic, roaring, etc.

SPEED: 5

Lightning quick, and with a tendency to shape-shift.

INTELLIGENCE: 5

As wily, cunning and clever as a four-year-old who doesn't want to go to sleep.

ACHILLES HEEL

Torches, cuddles, lavender spray.

Confirm or deny?

When faced with an imaginary creature, there are two schools of thought. Some firmly deny the existence of the scary thing, so children know there is nothing to fear, though this involves treating emotion with logic, which doesn't always work.

The other is to accept it as truth (after all, if we don't believe in wonderful, invisible things, how do you explain Santa?) but reassure them that you will sort it.

> 'It's no good just saying "there's no such thing". You have to enter their world. Say, "Show me the monster," then turn it round and say, "Oh look, he's just lost. Let's send him on his way." The monsters are symbolic. They just want to be believed.'
> *Spidermama*

Be warned, however: entering too far into the scenario creates its own problems:

> 'My dad took a wooden sword to the monster under my bed. Lots of groaning and swiping. He dragged it off yelling "don't look" over his shoulder. Backfired spectacularly as I didn't really believe there was one – except he'd obviously

caught an absolute whopper SO IT WAS REAL AND I BET IT HAD FRIENDS.'

Friskyhenderson

All this is general, though: time for specifics. Here are a few tried-and-tested methods to rid your child's bedroom of the entire taxonomy of night-time baddies.

Dragons, witches and other fairyland ruffians
Dragons are the most common type of under-bed squatter – and no wonder, given their prevalence in books and films. They're also an uncertainty: in some stories they're heroes, in others villains. There's a positive to this in that <winks conspicuously> you MAY JUST FIND that your particular witch or dragon turns out to be a GOOD one. . . However, should your child remain unconvinced, there are plenty of fail-safe ways to boot their scaly backsides out for good.

'My two-year-old is scared of dragons. But his Tigger is an excellent dragon fighter and we shout "BOO!" at them. He thinks this is great fun, and worries far less now.'

GeorginaA

Another method is to hurl a bit of treasure out into the front garden. Well-known for their love of gold, greedy dragons are certain to scamper after it. Make sure to yell 'And STAY out!' as they leave. Witches and wizards, meanwhile, are easily defeated in a number of ways:

'Sleep with a magic wand under the pillow. Witches can sense the presence of a magic wand and won't approach unless invited.'

Trucksanddinosaurs

'Pennies on the window ledge keep them away...'

Missnevermind

Monsters Inc.
These require careful treatment. Have a chat with your child first, and note any distinguishing features the monster has that will help you identify it. Many are much nearer the 'cheeky and naughty' end of the scale than the thoroughly evil. If you think you're dealing with a young monster, a gentle nudge might be all they need:

'I say loudly: "There are no monsters in here, are there? Because it's getting late and your mummy said it was time for you all to go home

to bed!" He loves the fact that monsters have a
mummy and a bedtime, too.'

Chinupchestout

For older monsters, a firmer approach is required:

'Try a few drops of lavender oil mixed with water
in a spray bottle. Monsters HATE lavender!'

Thereturnofthesmartarse

'We put dream catchers up to catch all monsters. Occasionally we take them down and
shake them outside because they're getting full.'

Notapizzaeater

A final word of warning on monsters: do be sure
you have correctly identified the species. . .

'On holiday our son kept saying there were
monsters under his pillow. The monsters turned
out to be mice when, a week later, my husband
lifted the bed and one ran out!'

Spottybra

Lions and tigers and bears, oh my!
Animal intruders fall into two camps: scary creatures from fiction (bears, wolves, tigers, etc.) and

utterly random animals that have unfathomably insinuated themselves under your child's bed.

We'll start with the first camp. Big cats are a more common occurrence under beds than you'd think (we blame Judith Kerr and her uninvited beer-swilling, sandwich-eating Tiger). Try lion poo (available from garden centres as a deterrent to cats). Spread liberally among your borders, it has the added bonus that, even once your tiger has left, the neighbourhood moggies will still leave your plants alone.

Unsurprisingly, wolves are common, and an absolute devil to get out from under furniture.

'My four-year-old is scared of wolves. I told him there are no wolves in England and anyway, the front door is locked. The next time he asked "What if they have keys?" I told them they couldn't get our keys and even if they did, their silly furry paws wouldn't be able to use them.'

Witchycat

With slightly older children, a little Gothic horror can work wonders:

'Nail a crucifix above their bed and tell them monsters and wolves are frightened of it.'

RosemaryWoodhouse

'Try lavender pomanders over the door. I drew
the line at garlic (used silver crosses instead,
I was NOT having garlic upstairs).'

Andro

Well, quite. If you've had a wolf through the
place, the last thing you need is any *more* noxious
smells.

Bears also loom large and are terrors for dig-
ging up carpet. Again, their prevalence is probably due to featuring regularly in familiar tales
(starving girls of porridge and turfing them out
of beds). If a scary bear in a story has triggered
the issue, combat it with a book about a friendly
bear. Paddington is always a good non-threatening
option, hard stare aside.

'We have a book called *Dear Bear* about a
girl who's afraid of the bear under the stairs.
Her parents write notes from the bear. Bear
invites girl to tea and he brings a note saying
he's lonely and would like to live with her.'

MrsApronStrings

Any similar plan that involves confronting the fear
during daylight hours might help them feel braver
at bedtime:

'With our daughter it was crocodiles. We played games in daytime where we were chased by crocodiles and successfully rescued each other.'

Eeemie

The more random, less scary animals actually require more initiative – but don't let lack of experience intimidate you. These Mumsnetters all found ingenious solutions to unwanted critters:

'Our son is frightened of walruses! He thinks they swim up the sides of his bed at night. We bought a toy walrus and we "wipe" the bed and anywhere else he suggests with it.'

busybusybee

'We keep a can of "octopus spray" (deodorant covered in parcel tape with a sticker on).'

Pachyclairbingobabe

Other homes suffer from much more pedestrian pests, though they are no less frightening to their victims.

'Our daughter became scared of badgers when we had cubs playing in the garden at night. Husband went out and had a loud conversation with the badgers – having left her bedroom window open. He told them nicely that she wanted

to go to sleep so would they please go away.
What the neighbours thought I don't know.'

Utka

Reclaiming territory from terror

Once you think you're rid of all pests, carry out a
test just to be sure:

'We put monster food under the bed (apples
and cat biscuits). If it isn't eaten by morning,
you'll know they've gone.'

Barbarianoftheuniverse

As with most childhood nasties, prevention is better than cure, so once you've beaten off the beasties, ensure defences are strong:

'My daughter (four) drew a "protective" monster and we stuck it next to her bed.'

Onceuponathyme

'I left the dog in their room for the night.'

Gibberthemonkey

Know when you're defeated

Now you can slay a dragon and turf out a tiger,
what of the bedtime beasts that defy all logic? If
you're plagued by any of the following we suggest you give the child a torch and a cuddle, retreat

downstairs, pour yourself a large drink and repeat the mantra 'this too shall pass'...

> 'Apparently there is a crab in our back garden, "crabbing". There are no crabs in our garden. There is no way a crab could be in our garden.'
>
> Butterpieify

> 'My son, now ten, used to be petrified of Sooty, as well as (wait for it) Sophie Ellis Bextor!'
>
> Shabster

> 'We are plagued by someone called "Mrs Wallace".'
>
> Soothepoo

Seriously though...
Teaching your child coping skills such as deep breathing or remembering a time they felt really happy will help them feel less anxious in general and is also a useful tool as they get older and fears of dragons turn into more rational concerns about the (still highly unlikely) possibility of burglary or fire.

Fear is a necessary part of development, so remember, during the wakeful nights, that while they're processing fear, they're learning the skills

that will keep them safe from real dangers through-
out their lives. Good night, sleep tight and don't let
the dragons bite.

AMAZING BEASTS-UNDER-THE-BED FACT
A 2013 survey of 2,000 parents found the most
common thing their children feared was spiders
and bugs (25%). Witches were the top fear of only
15% – less scary than clowns at 17%.

Postscript

No one said life as a parent would be easy. Nor did they make any promises it wouldn't be terrifying, messy, exhausting and involve more Marigolds and bleach than you'd ever hoped to encounter.

There are certainly moments when every one of us has found ourselves up to our armpits in something we'd rather never have encountered, be it nit lotion, an award-winning nappy or doing battle with a wolf in the wardrobe.

'But it's worth it.' That's what they all say, isn't it? For the warm head nestled in your neck, the tiny sticky hand in yours, the photographs of chocolate moustaches and the sight of them finally pedalling a bike without stabilisers or reversing nervously off the drive in your car for the first time.

We suspect that's not the case, though. Those moments aren't simply some wonderful accident that makes it all worthwhile. They are nature's way of ensuring you don't send the disgusting little blighters, and all the many and various nasties they are hosting, off to sea at the first opportunity. And who could blame you?

So firstly let's be thankful for Mother Nature who, as well as sending us parasites and pests, sent us enough good times to make us forget (and sometimes even do it all again). Secondly let's hear it for mothers everywhere, and particularly the Mumsnetters whose sound advice we've collated here, because there's no wisdom like the wisdom of those who have gone before us and still bear the scars. And finally, let's raise a glass to Mother's Ruin. For while there may be trouble ahead, while there's a stiff G&T with your name on it post-bedtime, you can face the music, snap on the Marigolds and dance.

Acknowledgements

Writing this book would have been quite literally impossible without the glorious users of Mumsnet, whose tips, tricks and tales of parasitic woe underpin much of what is covered. I'd like to offer thanks and manly arm-punches to everyone who has ever found a nit, spied a tapeworm or de-crusted a spot and then ambled on to Mumsnet to post about it (hopefully after washing their hands).

I'd also like to thank the experts at Dr Care Anywhere, for their strenuous efforts to stop us recommending anything dodgy. Any remaining errors are, of course, entirely our own work. Thanks, too, to the lovely people at Bloomsbury for even entertaining the idea that a book about nits could be a goer and Will at Janklow for ever-assured advice and patience.

Finally, gratitude and undying devotion are due to Iona Bower, for her charm and good looks. She's not a bad writer either.

Justine Roberts, CEO & Founder, Mumsnet

Disclaimer

The information contained in this book: a) is not intended to be, nor is it to be treated as, a substitute for specialist professional medical advice; b) is provided by the author and publishers as part of a reference publication only; and c) is to be used for general information and advice purposes only.

The author and publishers have i) endeavoured to ensure that the information contained in this book is accurate and correct at the time of going to press; but ii) make no representations or warranties of any kind, express or implied, about the completeness, accuracy, reliability, suitability or availability with respect to this book.

If you have any medical concerns about your child we urge you to consult your health visitor or GP as soon as possible.

Note on the Author

Created in 2000 by Justine Roberts as an online destination where parents could pool their wisdom, Mumsnet is widely regarded as the UK's leading online community for parents. It has over ten million monthly visitors.